25

Minutes to

Fit!

The Quick & Easy Workout Plan to lose fat and getting fit in less time than you think!

The home-based, one dumbbell or kettlebell workout for the busiest person in the world – YOU!

Roland Denzel, IKFF-CKT, Precision Nutrition-Pn1

Galina Ivanova Denzel, NSCA-CPT, RES

Fit Ink Publications

Thank you for reading!

To get updates, news, and info on new books and projects, signup for our newsletter at EatWellMoveWell.com/contact.

Roland & Galina Denzel

EatWelMoveWell.com

Praise for 25 Minutes to Fit

Hey Roland,

I read your book, and wanted to thank you for the inspiration! I started thinking differently about workouts and weight loss. I also started to realize my stomach is like a fuel cell, and overfilling it didn't lead to better longer miles. I now realize that eating several times a day doesn't matter. Now, its smaller, smarter portions with better, healthier foods.

I also started thinking about exercising. My busy schedule sometimes doesn't afford me the [gym] exercise that I should be making time for, however I found a few things from your book, thought smarter and it's all worked out.

Thank you for the inspiration and helping me think about working out differently! The next day I felt sore all over, and normally I would chalk it up to getting old, this time it was feeling the workout from the day before!

— Anthony

Hi guys. Thanks for writing the book. You know, I've had that dumbbell set in the garage for years, but I always thought I needed more than just that to workout. Turns out that my one dumbbell is a great workout!

I had to add more weight last week, by the way, but I've actually LOST more weight than I had to buy at the store for my workouts! I'm down 15lbs!

— Brad

Table of Contents

25 Minutes to Fit

No time to workout? Yeah, I hear you. I get that problem, too. Fortunately, I figured out a good solution for those times in my life when things are just too crazy. Is your life crazy, too?

Is this workout for you?

Probably...

Are you a busy guy or girl? Are you looking to burn fat? Are you new to the training game and wanting to put on a little muscle, feel better, stronger, and harder? Then yes, this program is for you.

The single biggest barrier that I hear when it comes to getting into shape is the lack of time. People are busy, and carving out hours per week to go to the gym is so low on the priority list that it's, realistically, never going to happen.

But, you've been lied to, both by the people who tell you that you merely have to walk more and by the people that point to bodybuilding magazines and tell you that you need to hit the gym 5-6 times per week.

Lies, all of it.

I remember, years ago, looking at my Palm Pilot 1000's crowded calendar and trying to find time to squeeze some gym time into that little screen.

Between the kids, work, church events, cooking, cleaning (yeah, right) and my commute, it didn't look good. There was no way that I could find the time to drive home to change after work, drive to the gym, workout, drive home, shower, all before dinner. ...and all of this FIVE OR SIX DAYS PER WEEK?!?!

Not going to happen!

...and it didn't.

But I did find a solution!

But I can't workout 5-6 times a week!

The first step was realizing that it's simply not necessary to train four, five, or even six times per week to get results. Successful training programs by the likes of Alwyn Cosgrove, Dan John, Zach Even-Esh, and Lou Schuler often utilize short and sweet workouts in which you train just two or three times per week. In fact, it's more effective to use a training plan that fits into your schedule than it is to squeeze the "perfect training plan" into an already too tight schedule; this is a recipe for failure.

My friend Dan John (CSCS, RKC, Strength Coach, Highland Games champion, etc.) is wise in the ways of the world, and that means he's equally wise when it comes to training; "If you can only workout twice per week, then find the program that will let you do just that. Don't set yourself up for failure by saying you can train 6 days per week and then only make 3 of the workouts. You'll never succeed that way. And it doesn't take that much to succeed."

Do you really need to spend an hour or more in the gym?

Absolutely not! While bodybuilders and professional athletes might actually want to spend hours in the gym, you don't have to. In fact, many studies have shown that trainees (like you) need far less gym time than fitness magazines tell you that you need to stimulate muscle growth, produce strength increases, and shed fat. It's not the time, it's what you do in the time you have that counts.

In order to be time efficient, this program is divided into four short "chunks," or four workouts. Each workout is designed to take only 20-25 minutes, including warmup time.

Let's talk training

Before we dive right into the workouts, let talk a little bit about the terms that personal trainers throw around so easily, like everyone knows what they are talking about...

Let's come to terms, shall we?

Before I drone on too long about the awesomeness and efficiency of this program, let talk terms. When I started my own fitness journey, I didn't know all of these terms, and had to ask, google them, or just nod along and pretend. I don't want you to have to do that, so I'll briefly cover some of the most common terms in the fitness world, most of which are going to be in this book.

Trainers, like Galya and me, also talk a lot in shortcuts, abbreviation and acronyms, so let's define some of this mumbo jumbo, shall we?

Workout – This is simply an exercise session. Some people mock "working out," and say we need to TRAIN. Whatever, if I go to the office and say "I trained last night," there will be mockery from the other direction. The words mean the same thing in this context.

Training – See Workout, above.

Upper body – Arms, chest, back, etc. This is a workout that targets these areas, primarily. There is plenty of overlap, so we don't get too hung up on which part is where.

Lower body – Legs, glutes (butt), hamstrings, etc. This is a workout that targets these areas, primarily.

Movement – An exercise, even if it doesn't seem like one. Is a stretch an exercise?

Weight – In exercise terminology, this is what gives you resistance. It could be a dumbbell or your bodyweight, which are the two primary weights used in this program.

Reps – the number of times you lift a weight in a row. Multiple "reps" makes up a set.

Sets – a set is a number of reps in a row.

Ladders – a ladder is a technique that's highlighted by small sets of increasing or decreasing reps. More on this in a minute!

Rest – the amount of time you're doing pretty much nothing in between exercises. Sometimes it's just taking enough time to switch positions, and other times it's prescribed rest, like "take 1-2 minutes to rest before moving on to the next exercise."

AMRAP – As Many Reps As Possible. Just like an All-You-Can-Eat restaurant, it's not really a good ideas to max these things out. Do as many as you can WITH

GOOD FORM and then stop. That, my friends, is As Many Reps As Possible!

ALAP – As Long As Possible. Like AMRAP, don't kill yourself. When you're close to failure, stop safely, especially if you have a heavy weight over your head!

Warmup – Movements that prepare your body and nervous system for the heavier weights to come. For most bodyweight and high repetition exercises, joint mobility and a few low rep sets get the body well prepared to lift safely. For heavier weights, where you are lifting close to your maximum abilities OR if you are very strong, warmup sets with increasingly heavier weights will be required.

The Ladder

Most of the key exercises use a concept known as the ladder. I don't know who invented it or named it, but it was popularized by Pavel Tsatsouline, a former Soviet Special Forces trainer, bodyweight training specialist, and Russian kettlebell master. Pavel's ladder is a technique designed to allow you to do more repetitions of an exercise by ramping up the reps within the set itself. Take a look at one example, below.

Ladder Example

Overhead Press, 1 rep left, 1 rep right

Split Squat, 1 rep left, 1 rep right

Overhead Press, 2 reps left, 2 reps right

Split Squat, 2 reps left, 2 reps right

Overhead Press, 4 reps left, 4 reps right

Split Squat, 4 reps left, 4 reps right

Overhead Press, 8 reps left, 8 reps right

Split Squat, 8 reps left, 8 reps right

This was just one ladder, or one set, using alternating mini-sets to provide just a short rest as you change exercises. If you do the math, that's 15 reps per exercise, per side; likely a lot more than we could have done if you'd been asked to shoot for 15 reps, straight.

One extra benefit – for most bodyweight and beginner exercises and weights – is that starting off with a low number of reps and working your way up allows the beginning of your workout to also serve as your warmup. This saves you even more valuable time. Of course, if you're pretty strong and can lift heavy, then an additional warmup is certainly necessary.

Warmups

Many of the workouts within this program are bodyweight only, and require minimal warmup.

Typically, for instance, a warmup for pushups is pushups, just fewer of them.

Some exercises will have you lifting somewhat heavier weights, and for those, a short and exercise specific warmup is needed. Typically, unless you are very strong, we recommend that you choose a weight that's about half of your planned weight, and use that for your warmup. Five to ten reps are usually enough warmup for this program, as the ladders take care of the rest.

Here's an example of the 'Warmup Note' that you'll see throughout the program:

Warmup Note*: Since the Two Point Rows use added weight that may become heavy, make sure to do a set of 5 with about half of your planned exercise weight during the warmup. If you plan to do Rows with 25lbs, then use a weight of 10-15lbs during the warmup, for instance.*

The workouts, the hows, and the whens

There are four workouts, and each is simply an upper body or lower body session. This system has quite a few benefits that help keep it short, sweet, and time efficient:

• Follow the workouts in order (one, two, three, four, one, two, etc).

• In general, I suggest taking a day break every two or three workouts.

• You only have to warmup your upper body for an upper body session and your lower body for a lower body session. This saves time over a non-specific warmup. In addition, the use of bodyweight exercises and smart exercise choice with Pavel's ladders make your workout start as you're warming up.

• Because you alternate upper body and lower body workouts, you can workout on back to back days if you want or need to. You can even workout up to four days in a row, since you will always give one half of your body a break on alternate days. I don't recommend training five days in a row, even with an upper/lower split workout plan. You need to rest sometimes!

• If you have the time and want to train upper and lower on the same day, you can. By combining any two consecutive workouts together you'll be doing a full body workout in one day. Make sure to take the next day off, because you'll need it!

• Because each workout is upper body or lower body only, you can do two workouts on back to back days while still giving your worked muscle groups that needed recovery time, but if you have the time, like on a weekend, you can still train your whole body in one day.

Your equipment

In order to keep this workout easily accessible, I've chosen to use mostly bodyweight exercises, and just a few exercises that use an inexpensive adjustable dumbbell. You can use almost any dumbbells, or a set of kettlebells if you have them. To keep things easy for those just starting out, I typically recommend CAP's adjustable dumbbell set, available on Amazon.com. I like these because it's easy and cheap to add extra plates down the road.

For information, see the Resources page at EatWellMoveWell.com/NoTimeToWorkoutResources.

66

"When you make exercise a regular part of your life, you will lose fat – primarily fat – and have a body that you're proud to show off once the fat is gone. In addition, your hard earned muscle will protect you against easy fat gain in the future."

– Man on Top: Lose Fat, Get Fit, and Control Your Weight for Life

99

Your workouts

Do these four workouts in order, using one of the example schedules in the last section. After you finish with workout number four, circle back to workout number one the next time. It's that simple.

Each time you go through the workout, you should be a little stronger, and get in a few more reps. Eventually, you'll have to look at making things harder or heavier, because you'll be too strong for the program as written, and that's a good thing!

A note about the charts that you are about to see... Kindles and Kindle Applications do not handle charts and graphs well, so I've converted them to a full page image for your convenience.

In addition, full workout charts are available at EatWellMoveWell.com/NoTimeToWorkoutResources.

You can download them and read them in Acrobat Reader or print them out to carry with you as you train.

Disclaimer

You must get your doctor's approval before beginning this diet and exercise program.

This book/ebook provides information that you read and use at your own risk. We do not take responsibility for any misfortune that may happen, either directly or indirectly, from reading and applying the information contained and/or referenced in this book/ebook.

The programs and information expressed within this book/ebook are NOT medical advice, but rather represent the authors' opinions, and are solely for informational and educational purposes. Please do not use the information in this book without first discussing your fitness, training, and nutrition plans with a qualified doctor or health practitioner.

The authors are not responsible for any injury or health condition that may occur through following the programs and opinions expressed within this book. The dietary information is presented for informational purposes only and may not be appropriate for all individuals.

Remember, consult with your physician before starting any exercise program or altering your diet.

Workout One

Upper Body	Movement	Weight Used	Reps	Sets	Ladders	Rest
Warmup *	Face the wall Ys	Bodyweight	10 reps	1 set	n/a	None
	Joint rotations	Bodyweight	10 per joint	1 set, each side	n/a	None
	Pushups plus	Bodyweight	10 reps	1 set	n/a	None
	Two point rows *		5 reps, w/ ½ weight	1 set, each side	n/a	None

Workout One	Movement	Weight Used	Reps	Sets	Ladders	Rest
1a	Plank to pushup	Bodyweight	Ladders, 2, 4, 8, 12	n/a	2 ladders, each side	1-2 min after 1st
1b	Two point Row		Ladders, 2, 4, 8, 12	n/a	2 ladders, each side	pair of ladders
2a	Waiter's walks		ALAP	2 sets, each side	n/a	1-2 min after 1st
2b	Side planks	Bodyweight	ALAP, per side	2 sets, each side	n/a	pair of sets

* **Warmup Note:** Since the Two Point Rows use added weight that may become heavy, make sure to do a set of 5 with about half of your planned exercise weight during the warmup. If you plan to do Rows with 25lbs, then use a weight of 10-15lbs during the warmup, for instance.

** ALAP = As Long As Possible

*** N/A = Not Applicable

14

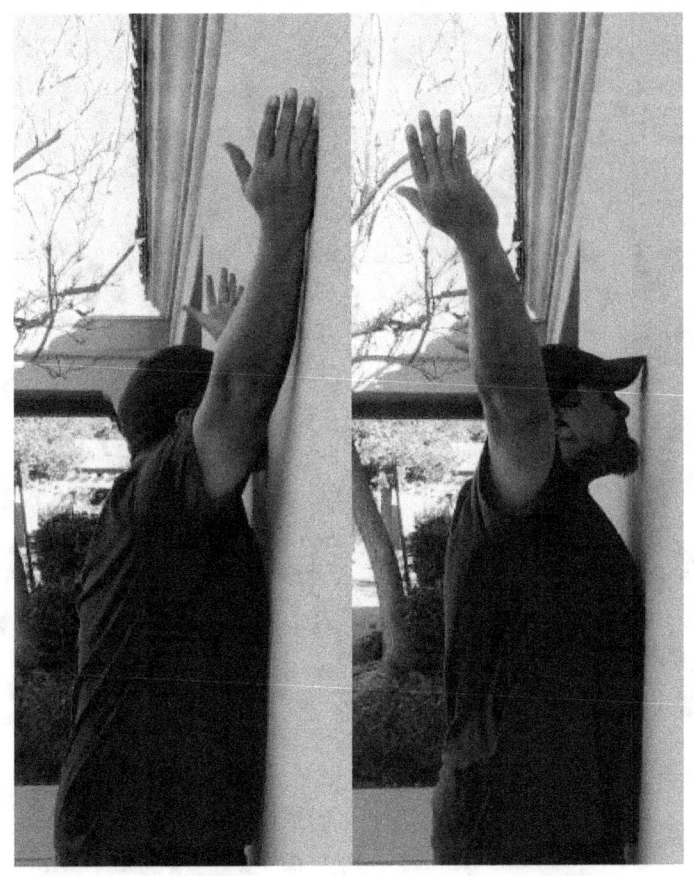

Face the wall Ys– stand close to a wall and stretch
your arms up and wide in the Y position. Keeping the
muscle between your shoulder blades tight, bring
yours arms away from the wall while keeping your
shoulders down and elbows straight. Hold for a
second. Bring back to start and repeat a total of 10
times.

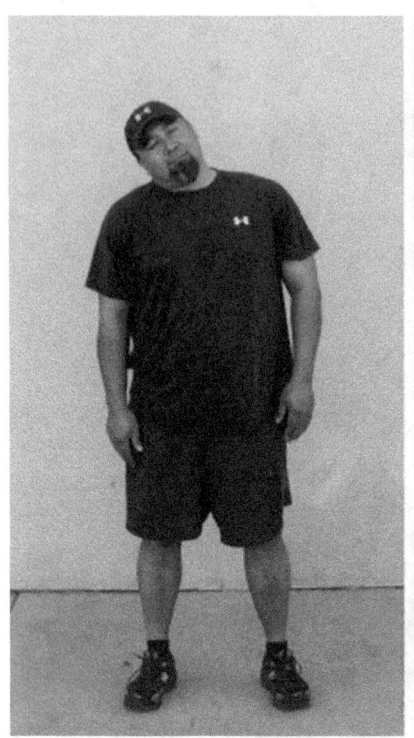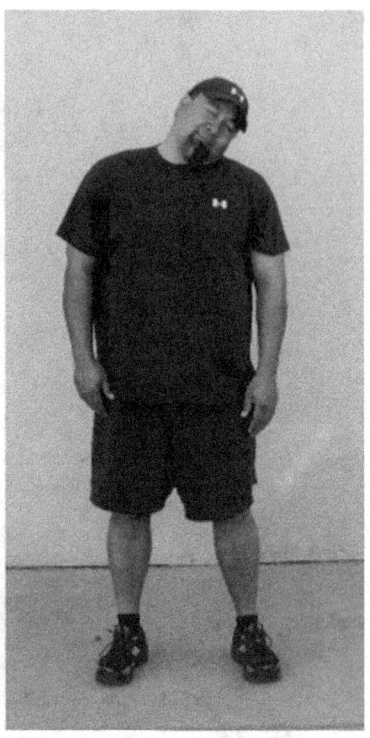

Joint rotations – rotate each or the major joints at least 5-10 times in each direction, starting from the top down: gentle neck rolls, shoulder circles, wrists circles, bending left to right at the waist, rotating your hips, bending your knees and rotating your ankles. This will disperse the fluid that lubricates the joints and ensure that no wear and tear occurs during workouts. It's an easy practice that yogi and martial artists have passed on for centuries.

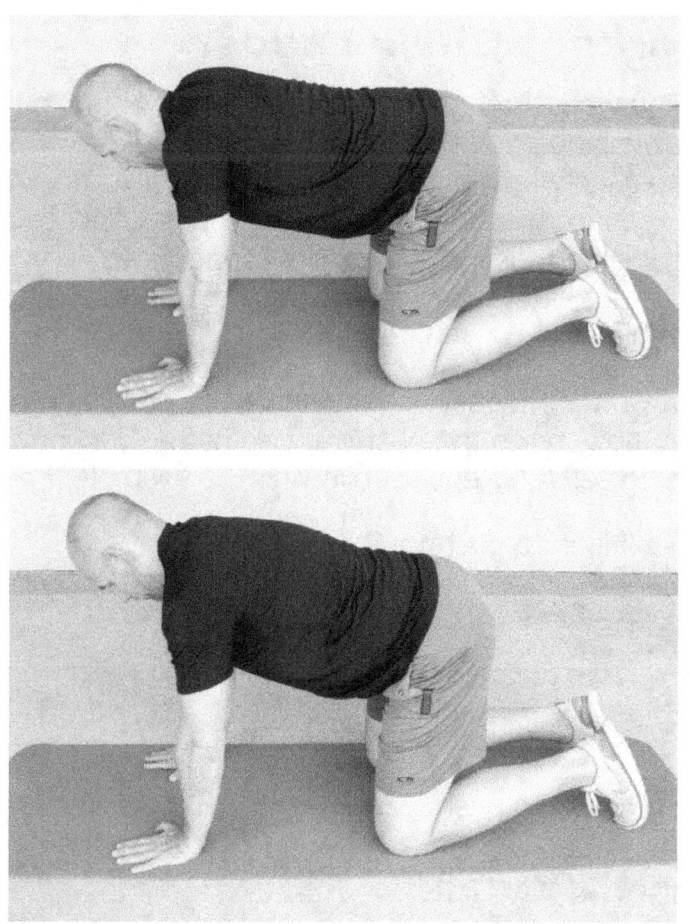

Pushups plus – Get down on your hands and knees and lock your elbows. Make sure that your low back is neutral and your abs are tight. Drop your ribcage down and let your shoulder blades come together. Keeping your elbows straight, push up with your shoulders so that your shoulder blades spread apart.

Do ten of these.

Workout One's Ladder

As you work through today's ladder, you're going to be switching back and forth between exercises frequently, which not only gives you brief rests between muscle groups (allowing you to lift more or heavier), but also acts a lot like cardio, keeping your heart rate high, your blood pumping, and the calorie burn big!

Perform the first set of each ladder for each side, then move on to the next exercise before coming back to set #2. Repeat, following the example, below:

1.   Plank to pushup, 2 R

2.   Plank to pushup, 2 L

3.   Two point dumbbell row, 2 R

4.   Two point dumbbell row, 2 L

5.   Plank to pushup, 4 R

6.   Plank to pushup, 4 L

7.   Two point dumbbell row, 4 R

8.   Two point dumbbell row, 4 L

9.   Plank to pushup, 8 R

10.   Plank to pushup, 8 L

11.   Two point dumbbell row, 8 R

12. Two point dumbbell row, 8 L

13. Plank to pushup, 12 R

14. Plank to pushup, 12 L

15. Two point dumbbell row, 12 R

16. Two point dumbbell row, 12 L

It's likely, and expected, that most people won't be able to finish the ladder at first. For many, the set of 8 might be where they hit a wall. It doesn't matter, because the beauty of the ladder concept is that they are self-limiting. Just keep track of how far you get from workout to workout, and watch as you get better and stronger!

Repeat this pattern until you've done all the reps of each set of the ladder WITH GOOD FORM.

After the first ladder is complete, rest for 1-2 minutes, then go back for your second full ladder.

When you can't finish a set within a ladder, just stop. Don't struggle to finish that set, just move on to the next exercise or side. If you have another set of that ladder to go, still do it when you come back to it, but only do what you can. One day, you'll complete all sets within the ladder, and then we'll have to worry about making things harder for you (insert evil laugh, here!). Until then, just get in your reps!

Repeat this pattern until you've done all the reps of the ladder you can do with good form. When you can do all sets of the ladder for all reps, it's time to consider adding weight or making things harder!

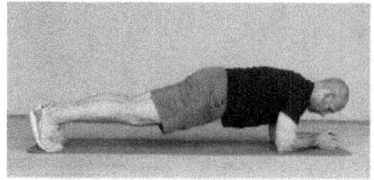 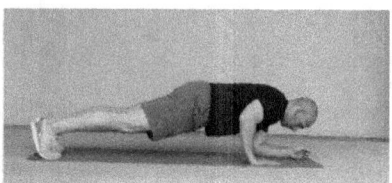
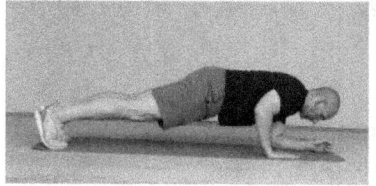 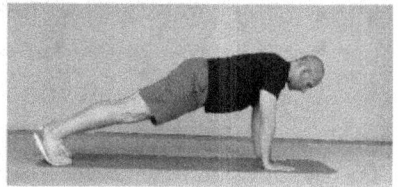

Plank to pushup – Get in a plank position on elbows and toes with your spine neutral and your head, shoulder blades, and hips in line. Keeping your abs tight, push yourself up with one hand, following with the other until you are in the top of a pushup position. Reverse the steps, dropping down to one elbow, then the other.

Watch the elbows!

To protect your elbows and forearms during the Planks to pushups, use a yoga mat, carpet, grass, or even a folded towel between you and the floor. If you do them straight on a hard floor, you'll be bruised up in no time!

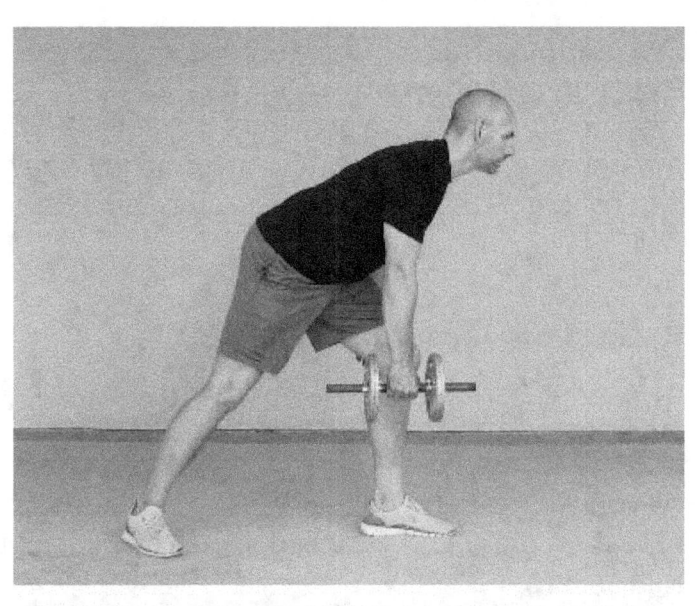

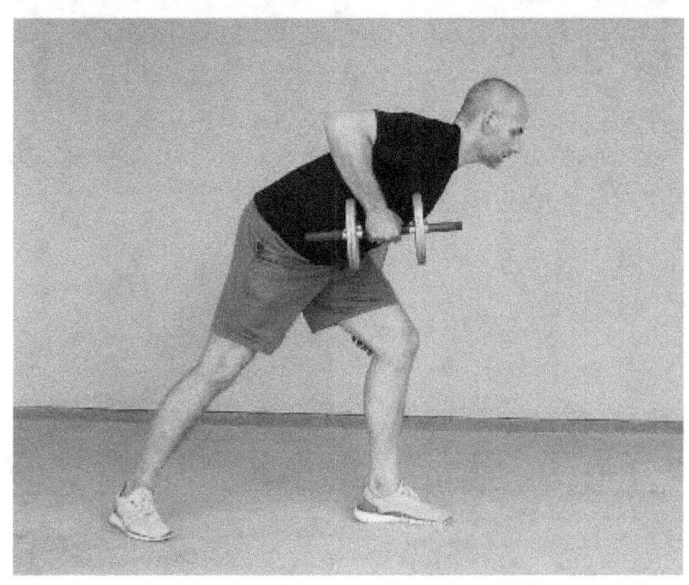

Two point dumbbell row – Take a split stance stepping forward with your left foot and bend over keeping your back straight. Hold a dumbbell with your right hand and row up, keeping your body straight and using the muscles between your shoulder blades.

Back to the ladder instructions...

Extend your arm back down and repeat for all reps of that ladder.

As you work through the ladder, switch arms and repeat on the other side. 1 Right, 1 Left, 2 R, 2 L, 4 R, 4 L, 8 R, 8 L

When you are completely done with all ladders, rest 1-2 minutes before moving on to the Waiter's Walks and Side Planks.

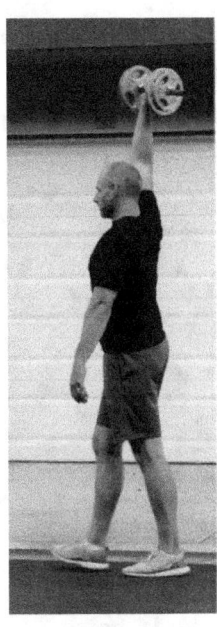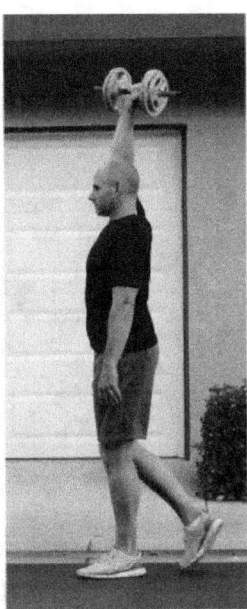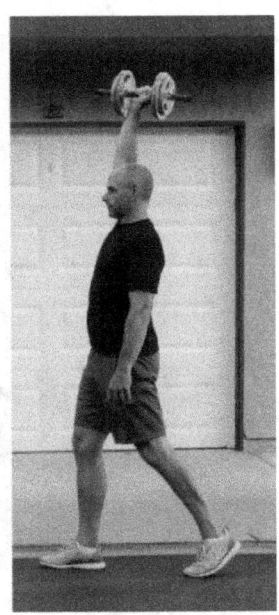

Waiter's Walks –Choose a dumbbell that you could overhead press at least 10 times for this exercise. Starting with your non-dominant arm, press the weight overhead. Making sure that your torso and hips are pointed straight, walk forward, keeping your shoulder stable. Walk slowly until your arm, shoulder, or core becomes fatigued, then carefully lower it to your shoulder.

If you can walk for over a minute without feeling challenged, then you probably need a heavier weight.

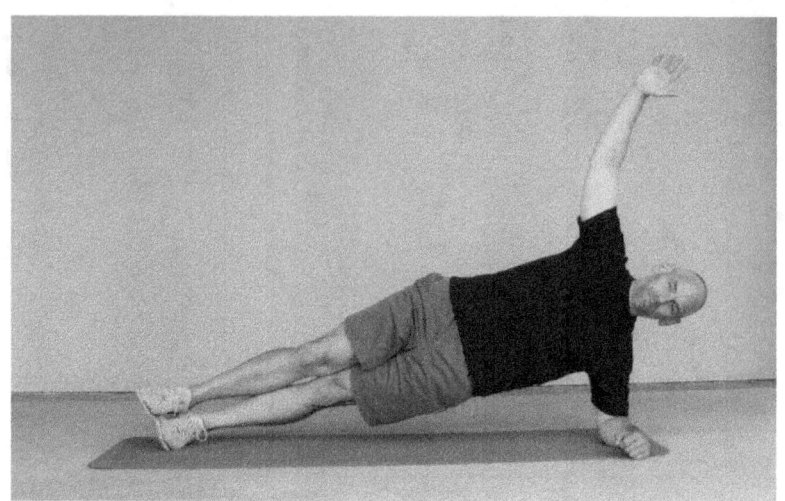

Side Planks – Lie on your side and place your elbow directly under your shoulder. Put your hips, knees, and ankles in line and push yourself up. Hold this position for as long as possible (ALAP) and then repeat on the other side.

If you are not ready for a full Side Plank yet, you can do them on your knees, as shown below.

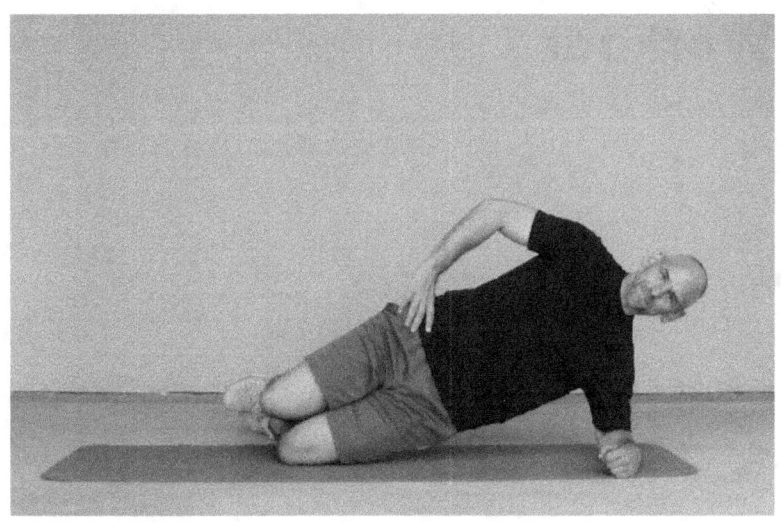

Side Planks, on knees – Lie on your side, knees
bent at a right angle, and place your elbow directly
under your shoulder. Put your hips and knees in line
and push yourself up. Hold this position for as long as
possible (ALAP) and then repeat on the other side.

Watch the elbows (again)!

*To protect your elbows and forearms during the
Planks and Side Planks, use a yoga mat, carpet,
grass, or even a folded towel between you and the
floor.*

Workout Two

Lower Body	Movement	Weight Used	Reps	Sets	Ladders	Rest
Warmup *	Split stance rotation	Bodyweight	10 per side	1 set, each side	n/a	None
	Ankle mobility	Bodyweight	10 per side	1 set, each side	n/a	None
	Glute bridge	Bodyweight	10 reps	1 set	n/a	None
	Split squat*	Bodyweight	5 per side	1 set, each side	n/a	None

Workout Two	Movement	Weight Used	Reps	Sets	Ladders	Rest
1a	One leg bridge	Bodyweight	Ladders, 2, 4, 8, 12	n/a	2 ladders, each side	1-2 min after
1b	Split squat		Ladders, 2, 4, 8, 12	n/a	2 ladders, each side	each pair of ladders

| 2a | Mountain Climbers | Bodyweight | 20-30 reps | 2 sets, each side | n/a | 1-2 min after 1st |
| 2b | Low to High Woodchops | | 10-15reps, each side | 2 sets | n/a | pair of sets |

* **Warmup Note**: If you're going to use added weight on the Split Squats, your warmup should include one set of 5 bodyweight split squats, per leg.

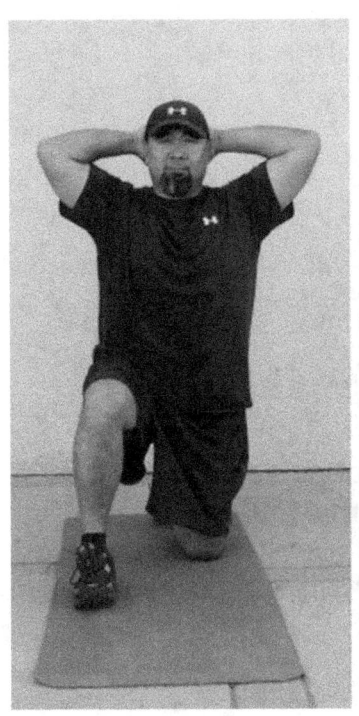 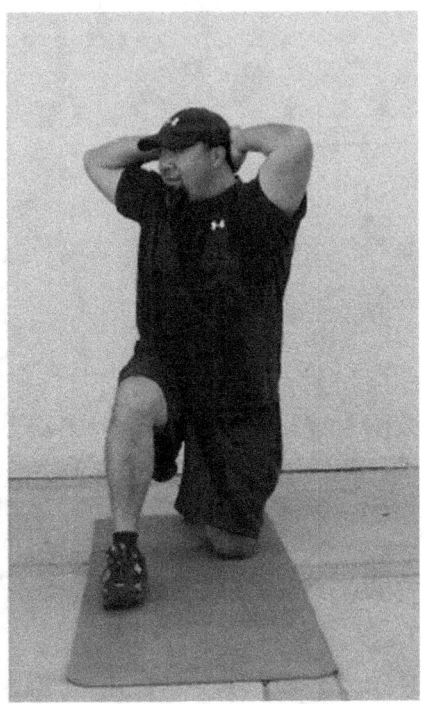

Split Stance Rotation – kneel down on one leg and put the other one in front. Stand tall and put your hands behind your neck. Keeping your elbows out, rotate towards the front knee and return to neutral., keeping your abs and hips in place.

Repeat ten times and then switch legs and do ten more.

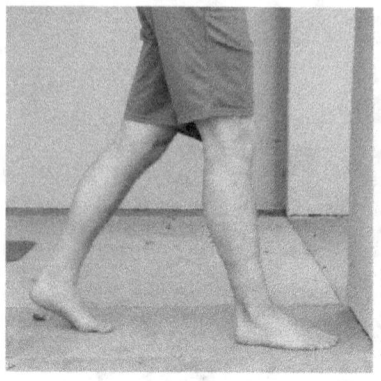 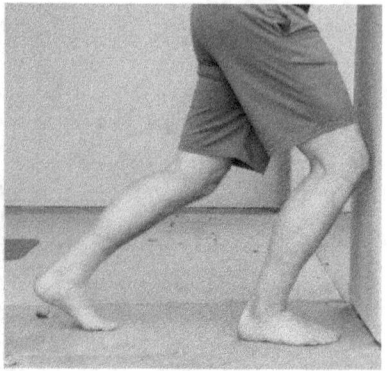

Ankle Mobility — Stand with your toes about six inches away from a wall and bring your other leg back. Shift your weight forward so that your knee darts toward the wall. If your knee can touch the wall, slide your front foot back another inch or so until you find it challenging.

Repeat for ten reps on each side.

Workout Two's Ladder

Perform the first set of each ladder for each side, then move on to the next exercise before coming back to set #2. Repeat, following the example, below:

1. One leg bridges, 2 R

2. One leg bridges, 2 L

3. Split squats, 2 R

4. Split squats, 2 L

5. One leg bridges, 4 R

6.   One leg bridges, 4 L

7.   Etc.

Repeat this pattern until you've done all the reps of each set of the ladder WITH GOOD FORM.

After the first ladder is complete, rest for 1-2 minutes, then go back for your second full ladder.

When you can't finish a set within a ladder, just stop. Don't struggle to finish that set, just move on to the next exercise or side. If you have another set of that ladder to go, still do it when you come back to it, but only do what you can. Repeat this pattern until you've done all the reps of the ladder you can do with good form. When you can do all sets of the ladder for all reps, it's time to consider adding weight or making things harder!

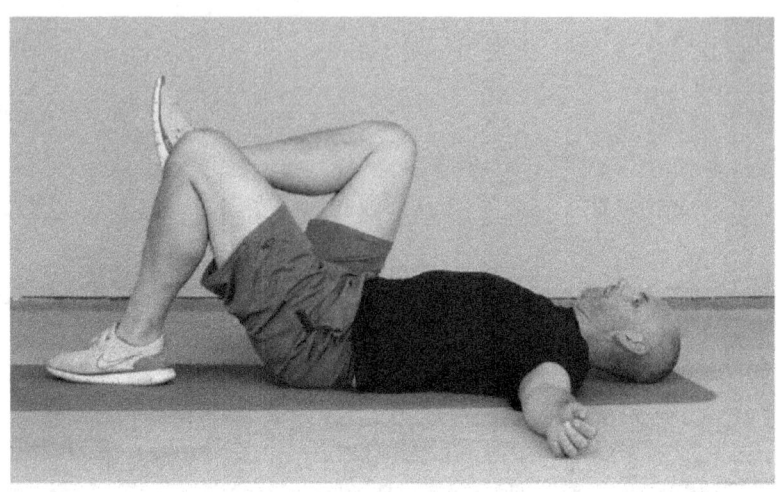

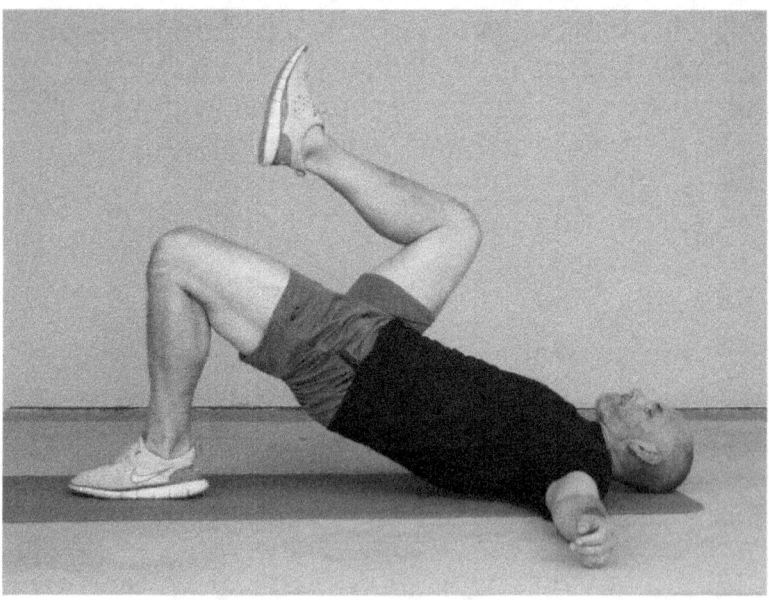

One leg bridges – Lie on your back and bend your knees. Hug one knee. Lift your butt off the floor, squeezing your glute as hard as you can and making sure you are not using the back of your leg or your lower back to lift yourself up.

As you work through the ladder, switch legs and repeat on the other side. 2 Right, 2 Left, then move onto the next exercise before coming back to this one for 4 Right, 4 Left, etc.

See the full description of how this ladder works in the description, above.

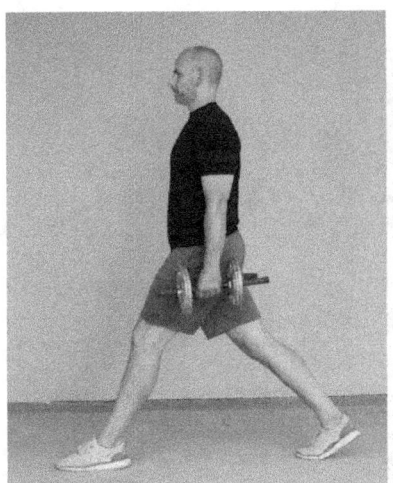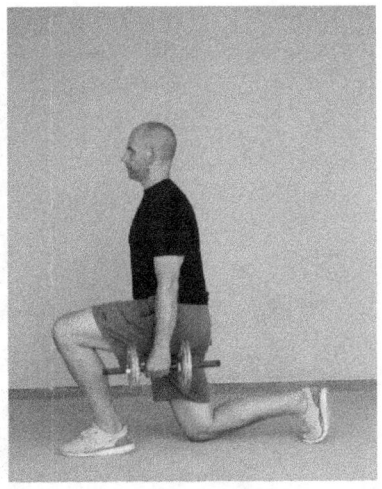

Split Squats – These can be done with weight or empty handed, depending on your strength. Using just one DB lets you focus more on balance and core strength.

Stand with one leg forward and with one or two dumbbells at your sides. Lower yourself down, until your knees reach 90 degrees. Push up through the front heel and return to starting position.

As you work through the ladder, switch legs and repeat on the other side. 2 Right, 2 Left, then move onto the next exercise before coming back to this one for 4 Right, 4 Left, etc.

When you are completely done with all ladders, rest 1-2 minutes before moving on to the Mountain climbers and Low to high woodchops.

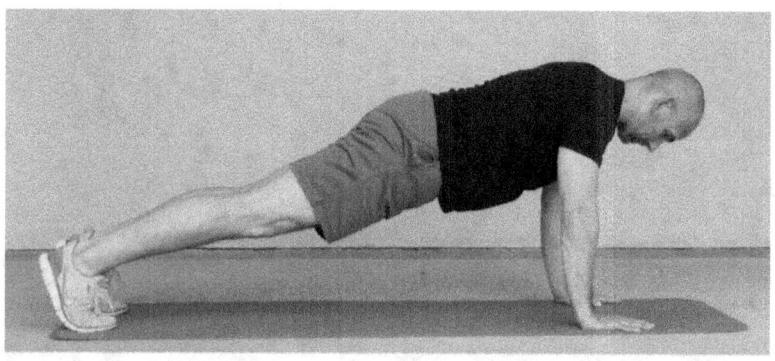

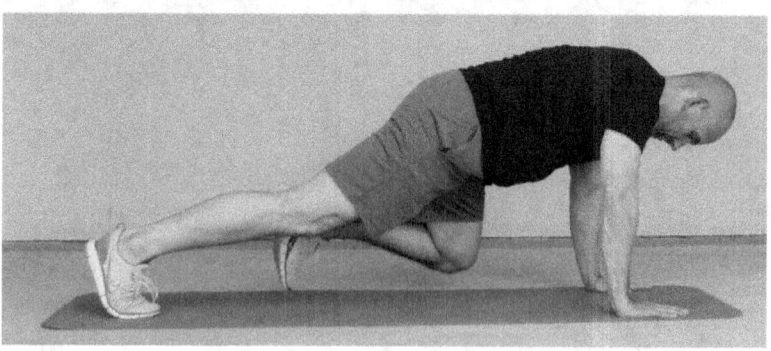

Mountain Climbers – Get in the top pushup position. Bring one knee to your chest and then return it to the starting position.

Alternating legs, bring each leg up to the chest and return to the starting position as fast as possible.

Do 20 reps (which is 10 reps per leg) before moving on to the next exercise, the Low to High Woodchops.

If 20 becomes easy, bump it up to 30, next time!

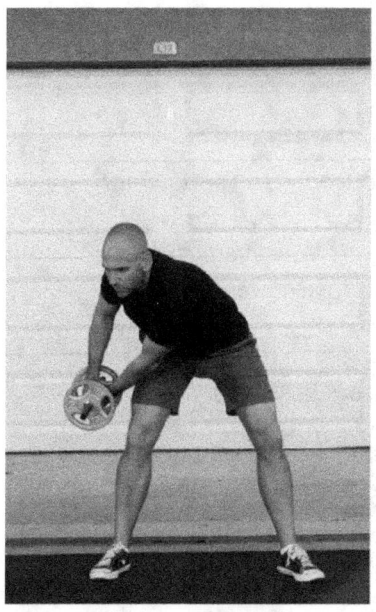
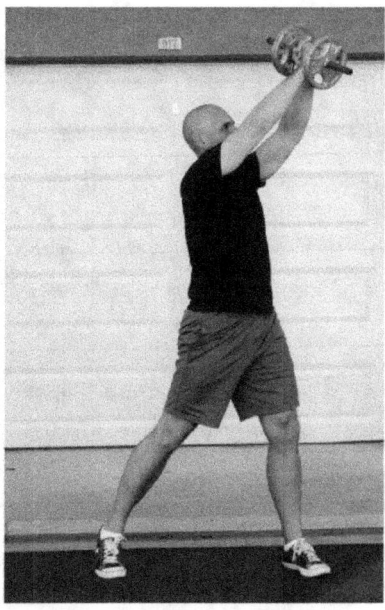

Low to High Woodchops – Hold one light dumbbell in both hands and on the outside of your right hip. Your feet should be slightly wider than shoulder width. Start by pushing your butt back as if about to sit in a chair. Do not squat down, but focus on pushing your butt back, assuming an athletic position. Contract your core muscles to move the dumbbell diagonally up and across your body, finishing with legs straight and the weight extended above your left shoulder.

Reverse the movement to complete one rep, then continue with all reps for this side before switching sides. Rest 1-2 minutes before returning to your next set of Mountain Climbers.

It's not about lifting heavy

> *With the Low to High Woodchop, you should not use a weight that's so heavy that you are straining to finish a rep. Start low, even using a jug of milk, medicine ball, or extremely light dumbbell.*
>
> *It's better to do a few more reps with a lighter weight than it is to use a weight that's too heavy and have to grind it out. It's about the movement, not the weight!*

Workout Three

Upper Body	Movement	Weight Used	Reps	Sets	Ladders	Rest
Warmup	Face the wall Ys	Bodyweight	10 reps	1 set	n/a	None
	Joint rotations	Bodyweight	10 per joint	1 set, each side	n/a	None
	Pushups plus	Bodyweight	10 reps	1 set	n/a	None
	DB presses*	½ weight	5 reps, each side	1 set, each side	n/a	None
	DB rows*	½ weight	5 reps, each side	1 set, each side	n/a	None

Workout One	Movement	Weight Used	Reps	Sets	Ladders	Rest
1a	DB presses		Ladders, 1, 2, 4, 8	n/a	2 ladders, each side	1-2 min after each complete pair
1b	Planks	Bodyweight	ALAP	2 sets	n/a	
2a	DB rows		Ladders, 1, 2, 4, 8	n/a	2 ladders, each side	1-2 min after 1st pair
2b	Pushups	Bodyweight	AMRAP	2 sets	n/a	

* **Warmup Note:** Since the Presses and Rows use added weight that may be heavy, make sure to do a set of 5 with about half of your planned exercise weight during the warmup. If you plan to lift with 25lbs, then use a weight of 10-15lbs during the warmup, for instance.

** ALAP = As Long As Possible, ** AMRAP = As Many As Possible

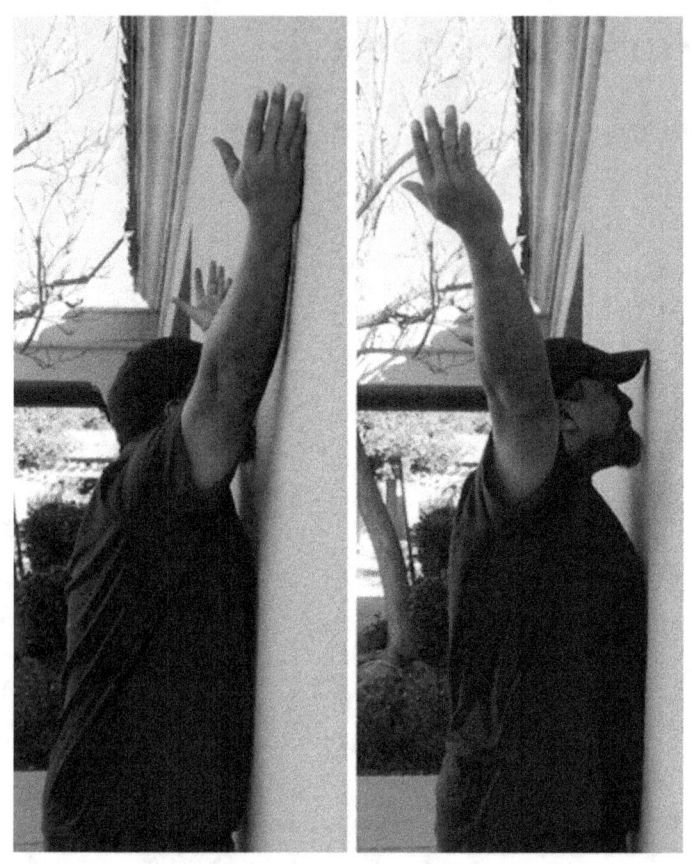

Face the wall Ys– stand close to a wall and stretch
your arms up and wide in the Y position. Keeping the
muscle between your shoulder blades tight, bring
yours arms away from the wall while keeping your
shoulders down and elbows straight. Hold for a
second. Bring back to start and repeat a total of 10
times.

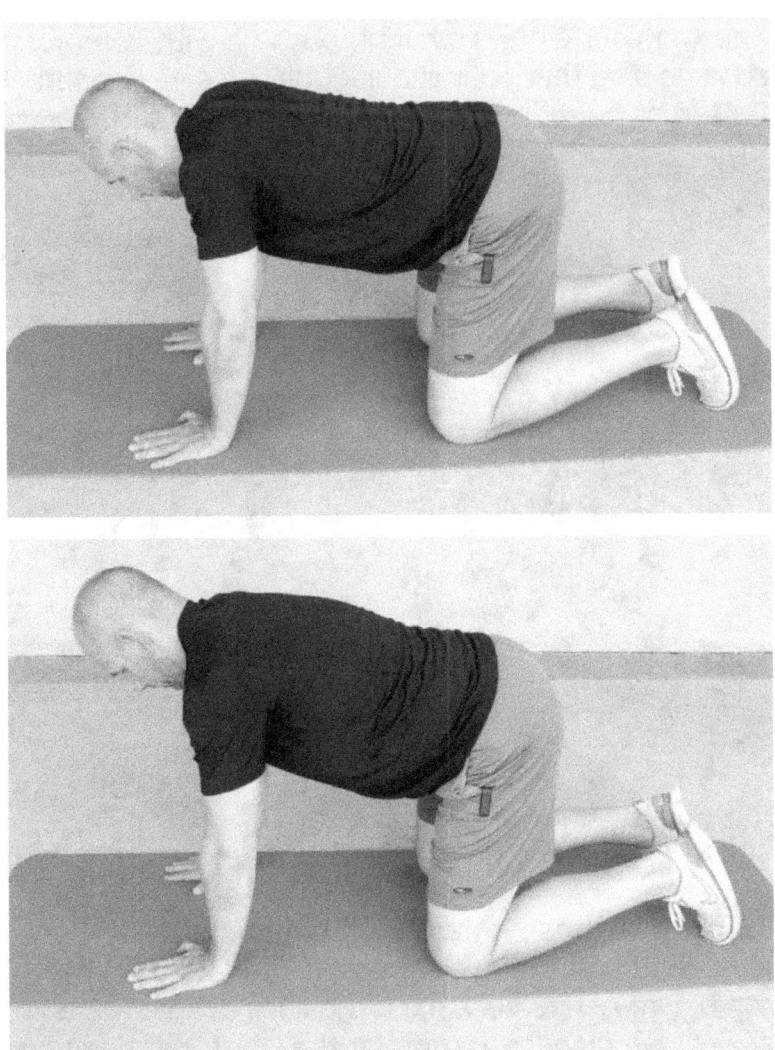

Pushups plus – Get down on your hands and knees and lock your elbows. Make sure that your low back is neutral and your abs are tight. Drop your ribcage down and let your shoulder blades come together.

Keeping your elbows straight, push up with your shoulders so that your shoulder blades spread apart. Do ten of these.

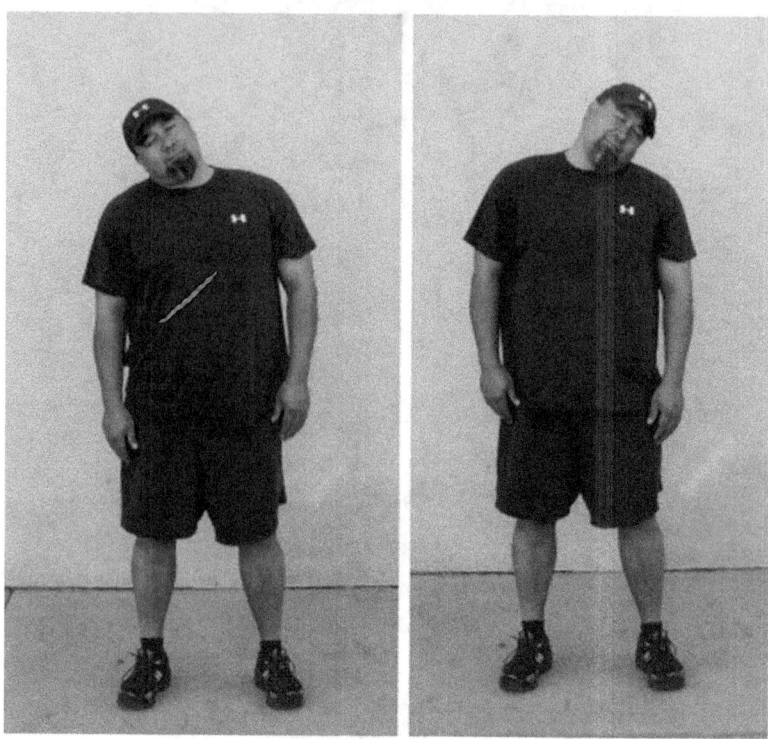

Joint rotations – rotate each or the major joints at least 5-10 times in each direction, starting from the top down: gentle neck rolls, shoulder circles, wrists circles, bending left to right at the waist, rotating your hips, bending your knees and rotating your ankles. This will disperse the fluid that lubricates the joints and ensure that no wear and tear occurs during workouts. It's an easy practice that yogi and martial artists have passed on for centuries.

Workout Three's Ladder

I paired each dumbbell exercise with a non-dumbbell movement so you can get away with just one dumbbell. I realize that changing weights around between each exercise is a waste of time, and that will not be tolerated!

Perform the first set of each ladder for each side, then move on to the next exercise before coming back to set #2. Repeat, following the example, below:

1.   Dumbbell Press, 1 R

2.   Dumbbell Press, 1 L

3.   Plank

4.   Dumbbell Press, 2 R

5.   Dumbbell Press, 2 L

6.   Plank

7.   Etc.

Repeat this pattern until you've done all the reps of each set of the ladder WITH GOOD FORM.

After the first ladder is complete, rest for 1-2 minutes, then go back for your second full ladder.

When you can't finish a set within a ladder, just stop. Don't struggle to finish that set, just move on to the next exercise or side. If you have another set of that ladder to go, still do it when you come back to it, but only do what you can. Repeat this pattern until you've done all the reps of the ladder you can do with good form. When you can do all sets of the ladder for all reps, it's time to consider adding weight or making things harder!

Ready? Let's see Workout Three's exercises!

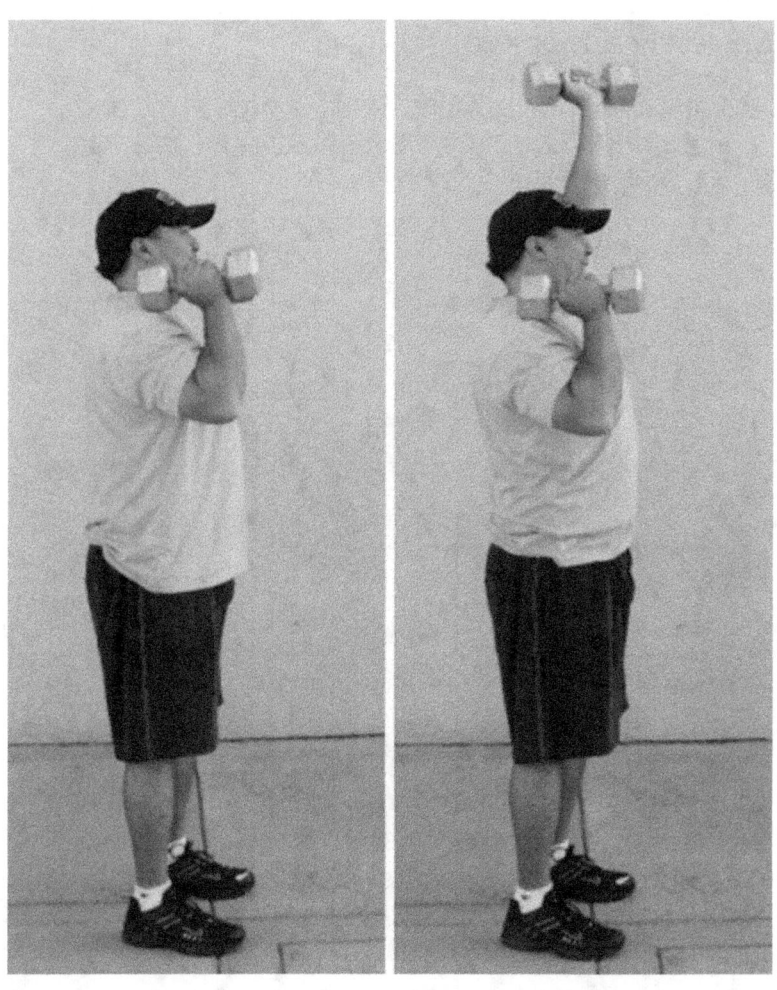

Dumbbell Press – Take a wide boxing stance, one foot slightly in front of the other, and hold a dumbbell at the shoulder.

Contract your shoulder blade to give your shoulder a stable support to push from and press the weight up, pause, and lower it under control.

Keep your abs braced the whole time.

As you work through the ladder, switch arms and repeat on the other side. 1 Right, 1 Left, 2 R, 2 L, 4 R, 4 L, 8 R, 8 L

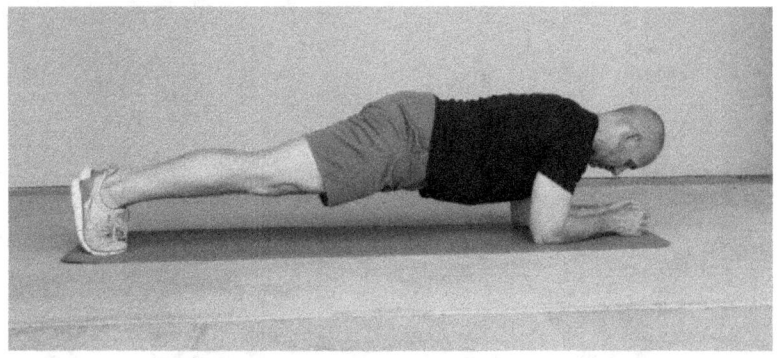

Plank – Get in a pushup position, and drop to your elbows, making sure your body is in one straight line from ankles through hips to neck. Do not push up with your upper back; rather focus on maintaining this position using your abs, all the while keeping your upper back neutral. Keep your butt cheeks tight and a straight lower back. Hold for as long as possible.

Note: If you are not ready for a full Plank yet, you can do them on your knees, as shown below.

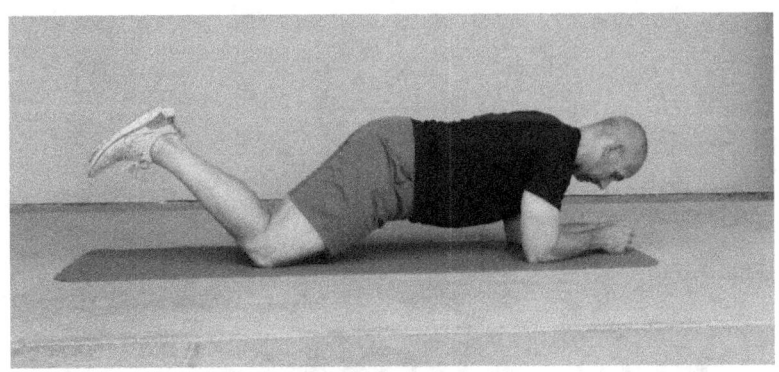

Plank, on knees – get in a pushup position, and drop to your elbows and knees, making sure your body is in one straight line from hips to neck. Do not push up with your upper back; rather focus on maintaining this position using your abs, all the while keeping your upper back neutral. Keep your butt cheeks tight and a straight lower back. Hold for as long as possible.

When you are completely done with Dumbbell Press ladder and Planks, rest 1-2 minutes before moving on to the Dumbbell Rows and Pushups.

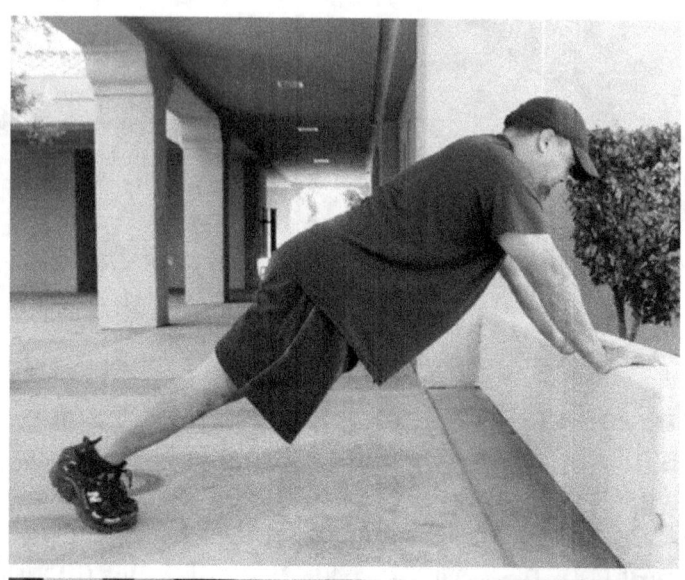

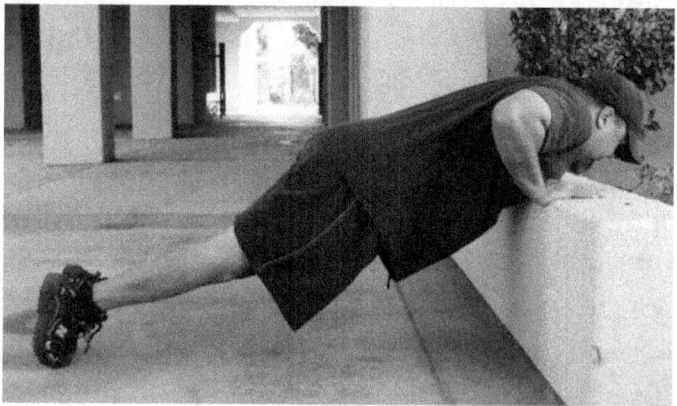

Elevated Pushups – Put your hands on a bench, chair, or wall, slightly wider than your shoulders. Straighten your body over the ground, rising up onto your toes. You will be at an angle, not flat over the floor. Keep your abs braced the entire time. The tighter your body, the more pushups you'll be able to do. Lower yourself until your chest is an inch or two from the bench or chair. Keep your body stiff and straight. Push yourself back up, pause, and repeat for as many reps as possible.

Because this pushup is done with hands on a wall or chair, it is a good choice for those who can't yet do regular pushups.

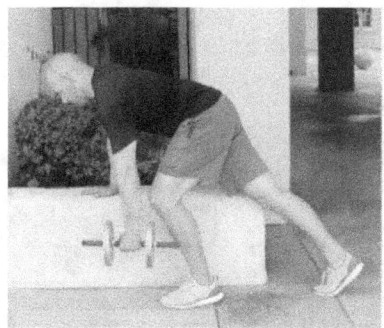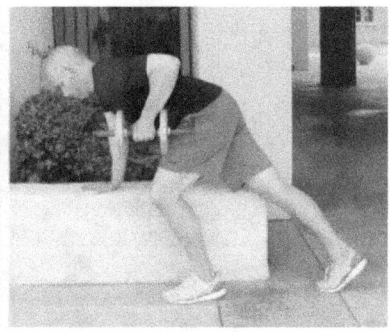

Dumbbell Rows – Assume a bent over position, with one foot slightly in front of the other, and the opposite hand resting on a bench, wall, or chair. Extend your free arm to grab a dumbbell, keeping your back neutral. Row the weight up using the muscles between your shoulder blades. Hold for a second and lower slowly, repeating for all reps for that ladder before switching sides.

As you work through the ladder, switch arms and legs and repeat on the other side. 1 Right, 1 Left, 2 R, 2 L, 4 R, 4 L, 8 R, 8 L

Workout Four

Lower Body	Movement	Weight Used	Reps	Sets	Ladders	Rest
Warmup *	Split stance rotation	Bodyweight	10 per side	1 set, each side	n/a	None
	Ankle mobility	Bodyweight	10 per side	1 set, each side	n/a	None
	Goblet squats *	½ weight	5-10 reps	1 set	n/a	None

Workout Two	Movement	Weight Used	Reps	Sets	Ladders	Rest
1a	Glute bridges		Ladders, 2, 4, 8, 12	n/a	2 ladders	1-2 min after 1st
1b	Goblet squats		Ladders, 2, 4, 8, 12	n/a	2 ladders	pair of ladders
2a	Jumping jacks/rope	Bodyweight	1 minute each set	2 sets	n/a	1-2 min after 1st
2b	Suitcase walk		ALAP, per side	2 sets, each side	n/a	pair of sets

* **Warmup Note**: Since the Squats use added weight that may be heavy, make sure to do a set of 5-10 with about half of your planned exercise weight during the warmup. If you plan to lift with 25lbs, then use a weight of 10-15lbs during the warmup, for instance.

** ALAP = As Long As Possible

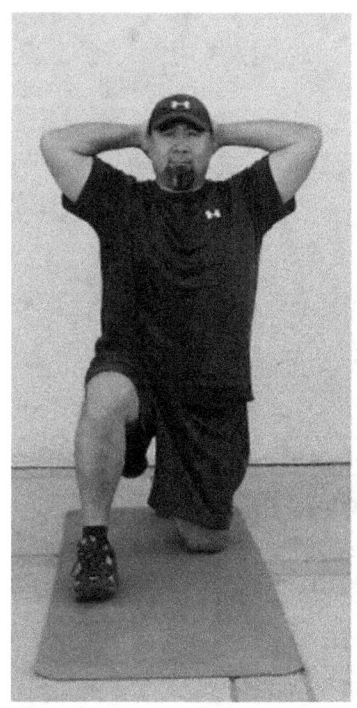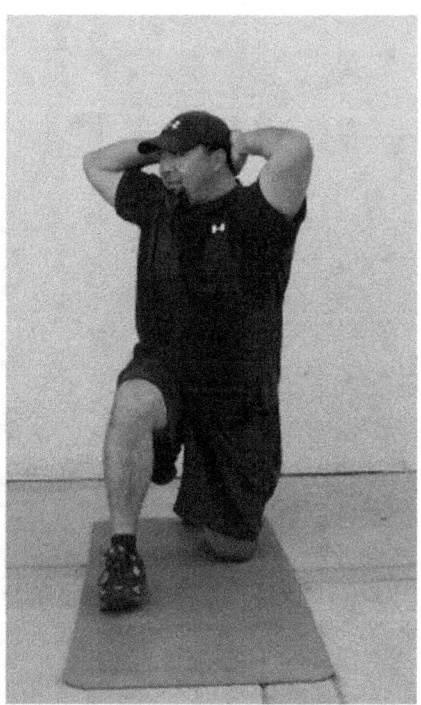

Split Stance Rotation – kneel down on one leg and put the other one in front. Stand tall and put your hands behind your neck. Keeping your elbows out, rotate towards the front knee and return to neutral., keeping your abs and hips in place.

Repeat ten times and then switch legs and do ten more.

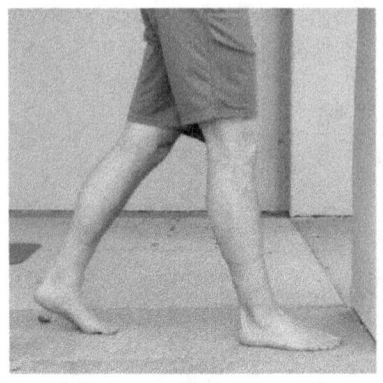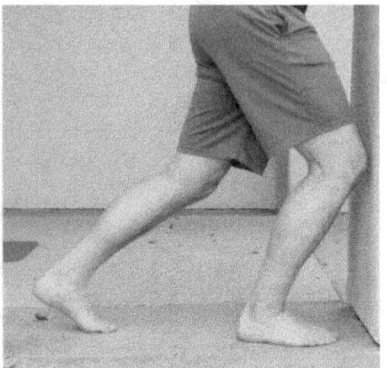

Ankle Mobility – Stand with your toes about six inches away from a wall and bring your other leg back. Shift your weight forward so that your knee darts toward the wall. If your knee can touch the wall, slide your front foot back another inch or so until you find it challenging.

Repeat for ten reps on each side.

Workout Four's Ladder

Perform the first set of each ladder for each side, then move on to the next exercise before coming back to set #2. Repeat, following the example, below:

1.   Glute Bridge, 2

2.   Goblet Squat, 2

3.   Glute Bridge, 4

4.   Goblet Squat, 4

5.   Glute Bridge, 8

6.   Goblet Squat, 8

7.   Etc.

Repeat this pattern until you've done all the reps of each set of the ladder WITH GOOD FORM.

After the first ladder is complete, rest for 1-2 minutes, then go back for your second full ladder.

When you can't finish a set within a ladder, just stop. Don't struggle to finish that set, just move on to the next exercise or side. If you have another set of that ladder to go, still do it when you come back to it, but only do what you can. Repeat this pattern until you've done all the reps of the ladder you can do with good form. When you can do all sets of the ladder for all reps, it's time to consider adding weight or making things harder!

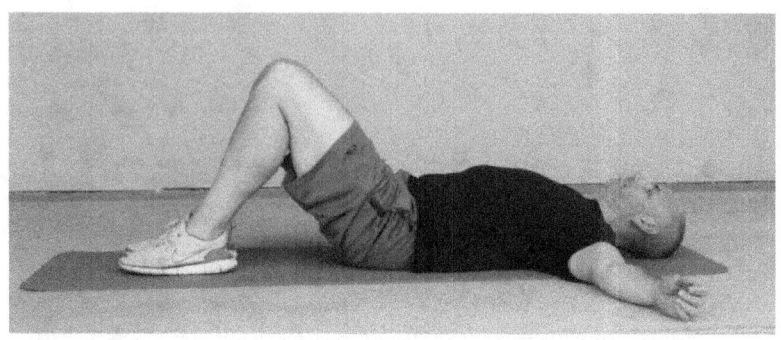

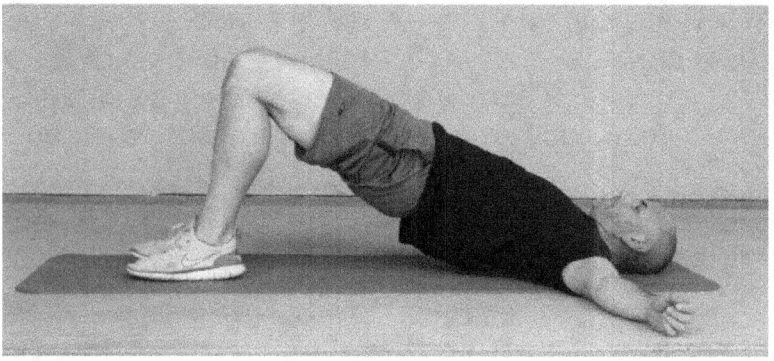

Glute Bridge – Lie face up and bend your knees. Squeeze your glutes and raise your hips off the floor forming a straight line. Do not use the back of your legs or your low back. Lower yourself to the starting position and repeat for ten reps.

As you work through the ladder, switch exercises after each set; 2 bridges, 2 squats, 4 bridges, 4 squats, etc. until that ladder is done.

Glute Bridges are too easy?

Some people get pretty good at these and they become easy. I you like, you can hold a small weight plate, medicine ball, cinderblock, or phone book on your lap as you do these.

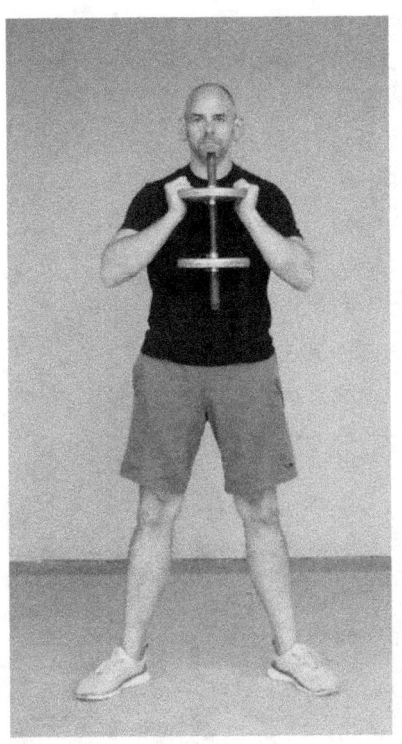 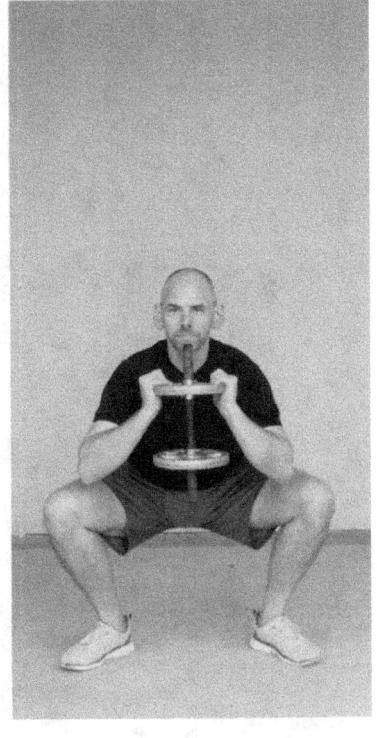

Goblet s Squats – Stand with your feet at shoulder width and hold a dumbbell in both hands at chest level. Sit far back until your thighs reach parallel, keeping your back straight. Use your glutes to push yourself up.

As you work through the ladder, switch exercises after each set; 2 bridges, 2 squats, 4 bridges, 4 squats, etc.

When you are completely done with all ladders, rest 1-2 minutes before moving on to the Jumping Jacks and Suitcase Walks.

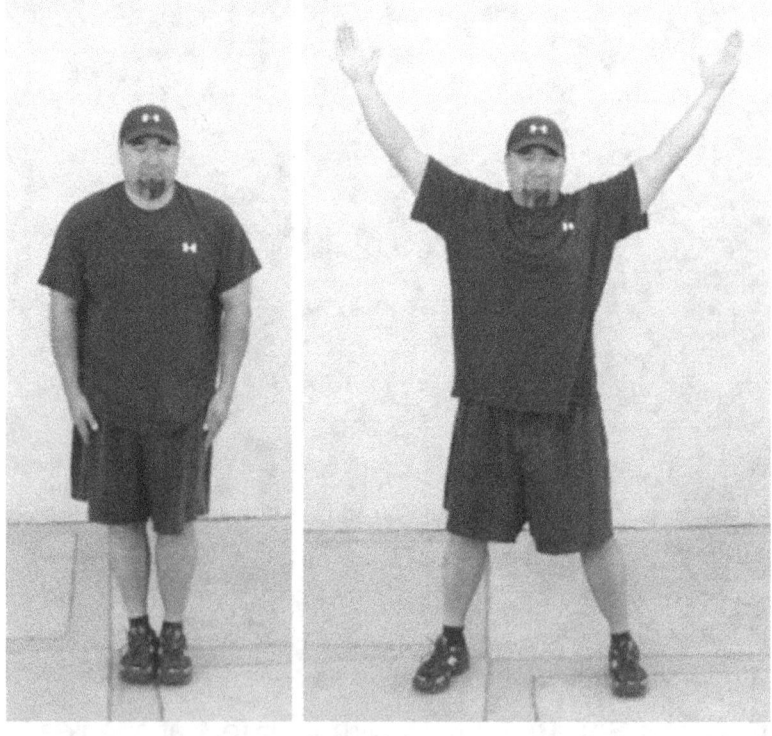

Jumping Jacks – Start with your feet together, hands at your sides. Jump and spread your feet to just beyond shoulder width, and simultaneously bring your arms up and together. Jump back to the starting position and repeat for one minute.

If you can't make it the full minute, note your time and try for longer, next week.

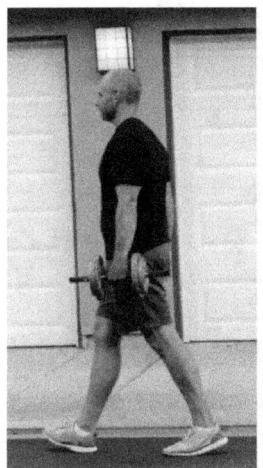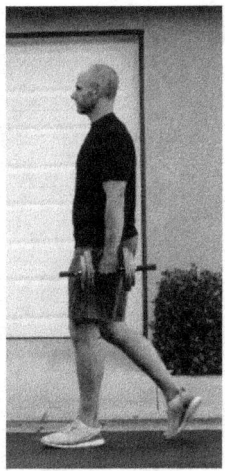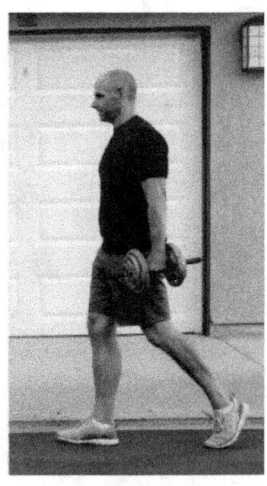

Suitcase Walk – Starting with your weak hand, hold a dumbbell of challenging weight at your side. Making sure that your torso and hips are pointed straight, walk forward as far as you can without losing proper form. If you can walk for over a minute without excessive leaning, or your grip isn't challenged, then you need a heavier weight.

Concentrate on proper heal/toe walking where you push off with your toes at the end of each stride.

66

"Eating better makes it much easier to eat less."

– Dr. Marion Nestle, Why Calories Count

99

Nutrition is half the battle

Or is it 70% of the battle? 80%? 90%?

Nutritionists, dieticians, personal trainers and doctors are all happy to share their ideas on what's important in the battle to get or stay lean. At one end of the spectrum, personal trainers want you to believe that following their programming is the key to great body composition, while some dieticians preach 'diet, diet, diet!' The truth, I assure you, is somewhere in between.

I'd love to tell you that nutrition makes up a specific percentage of your weight loss success, but truth be told, it doesn't matter what that percentage is, as long as you know it's big. I mean, if it's 70, 80, or 90%, what would you do differently? How do you apply that number to a burrito or slice of cheesecake? You don't, the math is too complex for mere mortals.

Good weight loss is a 50/50 partnership

Good weight loss? What do I mean by 'good' weight loss? Good weight loss means that primarily, excess body fat is lost, while muscle is preserved (or even gained). After all, if you lose 20lbs, and half of it was muscle, you haven't done yourself any real favors.

So, how do you prioritize your plan to lose fat and keep or gain muscle? That's where the 50/50 concept comes in. Don't worry about the exact numbers, but realize that each have to play their roles in order to be successful, just like with any good partnership.

Let's look at the part that each, diet and exercise, can play in your success. Let's look at the role of exercise, first:

• A weight training plan that progressively gets you stronger triggers your body to keep the muscle it already has, AND adds *more* muscle whenever possible.

• Exercise burns calories, whether it's cardio, aerobics, walking, or lifting weights. All exercise burns calories, and a smart weight lifting plan can actually burn *more* calories than most people's cardio ever will

• Resistance training increases your metabolic 'burn,' even after your gym time is over. When you lift weights, the training effect isn't over when you hit the showers, it continues on for hours, if not days. Haven't you ever still been sweating, hours after you've showered? Those are calories burning, baby!

• Recover is key after lifting weights, and recovery burns calories. Calories that you burn recovering are calories that you don't have to worry about *not* eating.

• Hard exercise leaves a lingering feeling of progress, even when that feeling is soreness. That feeling tends to remind us that we are working toward a goal, whether it's fat loss, muscle gain, or both. That reminder helps many people keep on track with their diet, since no one wants to feel like they just wasted their workout by eating away any progress.

You can't outrun a donut

"You can't out-train a bad diet" and "you can't outrun a donut" are two commonly tossed around phrases in the fitness and training communities, and they are largely true. You have to eat to support your training, not train to support your eating.

We just looked at some of the benefits of exercise, so now let's take a look at the nutrition side of things. What does nutrition – or your diet – do that exercise alone, can't?

• A good diet is one that provides good nutrition and high satisfaction levels, all while keeping calories lower. It's not enough to just eat less; not if you want lasting results, at least. The slogan of "eat less and move more" has been a failed attempt at fat loss and obesity control. Since USDA has started promoting the concept of "eat less, move more," obesity rates have only increased.

• A good diet is one that contains adequate protein, healthy fats, and just enough quality carbs to fuel your daily needs.

• A diet of healthy, whole foods is one that optimizes hormones and channels its nutrition to support your muscle mass, while eating away at unwanted fat stores.

• You don't have to count calories, but calories DO count. If you eat more calories than you burn, you're

58

going to store something; fat or muscle. If you want to lose weight, you HAVE to find a way to eat less than you burn, which forces your body to burn fat (i.e., stored calories).

• A good diet fuels your workouts. The better your workout, the more or heavier you lift. The more or heavier you lift, the more muscle you end up building. The more muscle you build, the more likely you are to lose fat when you *do* lose weight.

If you're already eating pretty well, then this program might be all it takes to let you burn a little fat or build a little muscle, but if you need more than that, keep in mind that you need to find a way to burn more than you eat to lose fat and you need to eat more than you burn to build muscle, so eat appropriately for your goal.

For good health and weight management, focusing on whole foods, quality proteins, healthy fats, and minimal carbohydrates is a good start.

Here are a few resources for more dietary and nutrition help. Links to all of the following resources can be found this book's resources page: EatWellMoveWell.com/notimetoworkoutresources

Our 30 Days of Real Food program is a 30 day 'reset,' designed to reset your dietary priorities, leave you slimmer, and healthier. It focuses on nutrient dense foods, and eliminates the foods that aren't the best for your health and waistline. The program is free, and available at EatWellMoveWell.com/30Days

Our Good Guys, Bad Guys page has the common ingredients and foods to focus on OR minimize during your quest for better health or fat loss. The page is in handy links on the

Our book, Man on Top is our complete system on managing your life and getting healthy, strong, lean, and fit. Man on Top is written using the same techniques and training that we use with our own clients; no gimmicks, no extreme diets, and just like with the book you're reading now, you won't have to live in the gym!

Links to all of the above resources can be found at:

EatWellMoveWell.com/notimetoworkoutresources

Time-saving, calorie-burning tips

I used to be single, childless, have a 9-5 job, and no one cared if my house was a mess.

Today, I have kids, a wife, a 9-5 (sometimes 7 to 6) job, clients, web sites to manage, books to write, and parents who need me. ...and trust me, people care if my house is a mess!

It's all I can do to find time to workout, make my food, and keep my training in check, but over the years, I've come up with a few tips and strategies to keep things on track. Take a look:

• **Workout before you shower** – If you workout at home, there's no one to smell you but you, so don't shower before you train (I was surprised to find out just that many people *do*). I'm sure you're not that stinky, anyway... Only showering once a day saves time, money, and water, which is in short supply in the United States, these days.

• **Organize your 'stuff'** – Once a week, right after laundry is done, organize all your workout clothes for the week; planning for five workouts a week? Make five stacks of shirts, shorts, socks, and underwear, plus any cool headbands or sweat towels necessary to keep you dry.

• **Make on emergency ~~supply~~ workout kit** – Depending on where you live, I'm sure you have an earthquake kit, a hurricane supplies bag, or a zombie apocalypse survival plan, but do you have an emergency workout kit? Not likely, and before I had one, I missed quite a few workouts because I forgot my gym bag, or even just one important item from the bag (you might be willing to train commando, but you can't train in dress shoes!).

Before you throw away those ratty old gym clothes that your wife or girlfriend is threatening to throw out for you, stick them in a bag and put them in the trunk of your car, just in case. I keep a pair of shoes, socks, underwear, shorts, shirt, and a large sweat towel. I go with the large sweat towel because it can work as an actual towel in a pinch, should I need to shower and head back to work!

• **Walking IS exercise** – It's not a substitute for strength training or high intensity training, but once you've done 2-3 days a week of weights and /or sprints, it's okay to take long walks, instead. Make it a point to walk TO the store instead of merely AT the store. Our grocery store is about ¾ miles away, Galya and I make it a point to walk there about twice a week. Driving wastes gas, burns fewer calories, and tends to make shopping a solitary experience.

• **Walking is an IMPORTANT exercise** – It's important that you realize that walking is as important as lifting weights, calisthenics, jogging, skipping rope, and swimming when it comes to calorie burn. In fact, once you've performed 2-3 weight training or resistance workouts a week, walking may be more important to your health than any other cardio workout. It requires no equipment, is safer on the joints, and doesn't cause the stress and need for recovery that more intensive exercise requires.

• **Housework & Yard Work ARE exercise** – If you don't have time to actually workout, keep in mind that more calories are burned by most household chores than by what we typically consider exercise. Housework and yard work is right up there with walking when it comes to its importance. In fact, since you HAVE to do it anyway, rank it higher. Work first, then walk; clean your way to the cleanest house in the neighborhood and the fittest you've ever been!

• **Recognize that more isn't always better** – I'm talking to those of you who start eating poorly just because they aren't training EVERY day. Do you try to hit the gym 5-6 times a week, just so you stay on your diet? Yikes. Not good, but I realize that some people are like that, and it really comes down to mindset; working out makes them conscious of what they eat. It also makes them less likely to go off the eating plan because they don't want to waste their training by eating badly and wiping out any progress. Change your idea of what working out really is. Eating right is just as important, if not more important, than burning 200 calories doing yet more exercise.

• **Mindset is important** – If you're having trouble considering regular day-to-day activities to be exercise, put on your workout clothes, crank up the iPod, and work up a sweat. This stuff IS exercise, so do what you need to do to make it seem like exercise!

The time is now, but I only have a few minutes...

> *A couple of years ago, Zach Even-Esh introduced me to the concept of breaking down workouts into more manageable portions, so there's always time to fit them into the daily grind. "Chunking," as Zach calls it, seems like a pretty obvious concept now, but back then, there was a belief in the fitness world that a workout needed to be forty-five minutes to an hour of hard work if you wanted to produce what we called the "anabolic window." Well, it turns out that your body doesn't care about any "windows," just that you do the work!*
>
> *Getting the work done makes sense, since our big and strong blacksmith and farmer ancestors didn't work the chest hard for an hour, drink a post-workout shake, take an ice bath, and then rest up until leg day. No, they worked when there was work to be done, and rested until they needed to work again. They got strong, and they built muscle!*
>
> *This program is designed to work in this same spirit, only instead of working out when you need to, you'll train when you can find the time.*

FAQ

Answers to the most frequently asked questions

We hope that the workout instructions are clear, but just in case, we've compiled the answers to the most common questions, and listed them below:

• Yes, just follow the workouts in order (one, two, three, four, one, two, etc).

• In general, I suggest taking a day break every two or three workouts.

• There are four workouts, and each is simply an upper body or lower body session. The four workouts are followed and repeated in sequence (One, Two, Three, Four, One, etc.).

• Yes, you only have to warmup your upper body for an upper body session and your lower body for a lower body session. This saves time over the traditional treadmill, non-specific warmup. Since we use a lot of bodyweight exercises, and choose strategic exercises and techniques (like the ladder) you're actually warming up even as you start to workout.

• Yes, because you alternate upper body and lower body workouts, you can workout on back to back days if you want or need to. You can workout up to four days in a row, since you will always give one half of your body a break on alternate days.

• No, I don't recommend training five or more days in a row, even with an upper/lower split workout plan. You need rest to recover.

• If you have the time and want to train upper and lower on the same day, you can. By combining any two *consecutive* workouts (one and two, three and four, four and one, two and three, etc.) together you'll be doing a full body workout in one day.

• Because each workout is upper body or lower body only, you can do two workouts on back to back days while still giving your worked muscle groups that needed recovery time, but if you have the time, like on a weekend, you can still train your whole body in one day.

• When doing upper and lower body workouts on separate days, train at least 3 days per week, but no more than 5.

• If you can't train 3 days per week, consider 2 days, but try to make at least one of you training days full body days, where you perform an upper and lower body session in the same day.

• If training twice on the same day, it's okay to do one session in the a.m. and one session in the pm.

- If you do two sessions in one day, allow yourself at least one day of rest before training again.

- Never skip a session (going from A to C, for example). Always alternate from an upper body day to a lower body day to an upper body day (A to B, B to C, C to D, D back to A).

- Workout a maximum of five days per week. Rest = recovery, and muscle is built during recovery, not during the workout.

- The schedule really is a simple as doing the workouts in order (one, two, three, four, one, two, etc.). When you consider your days off, it might look like this: one, two, three, break, four, one, break, two, three, four, break, one, etc.

- Yes, you *can* do more if you have more time, but if you have more time, why are you doing the No-Time-To-Workout Workout? ;)

If you have questions not answered here, please let us know.

Our full contact information is at the end, but you can always contact Roland by email at rdenzel@gmail.com.

...and what's next?

Of course, no training plan works forever; one day you'll hit a plateau or simply want to change up your program. Be ready for it, and plan ahead. I advise all my clients, family, and friends to always have a next plan. It's kind of funny to call it Plan B, but in reality It's just your next step in your training.

Read, whether it's books, blog posts of trainers you like, or stay Facebook friends with the best in the business. If you need advice on a next step, you can find us via email, on TheFitInk.com, through Twitter, and on Facebook!

We all, *always*, need to have a next step!

What's your Plan B?

Printable Logs

Remember, printable logs and links to other resources are located at:

EatWellMoveWell.com/NoTimeToWorkoutResources

The Authors

Roland Denzel, IKFF-CKT, Precision Nutrition-PnC

"Hi, I'm Roland Denzel, and I used to be fat."

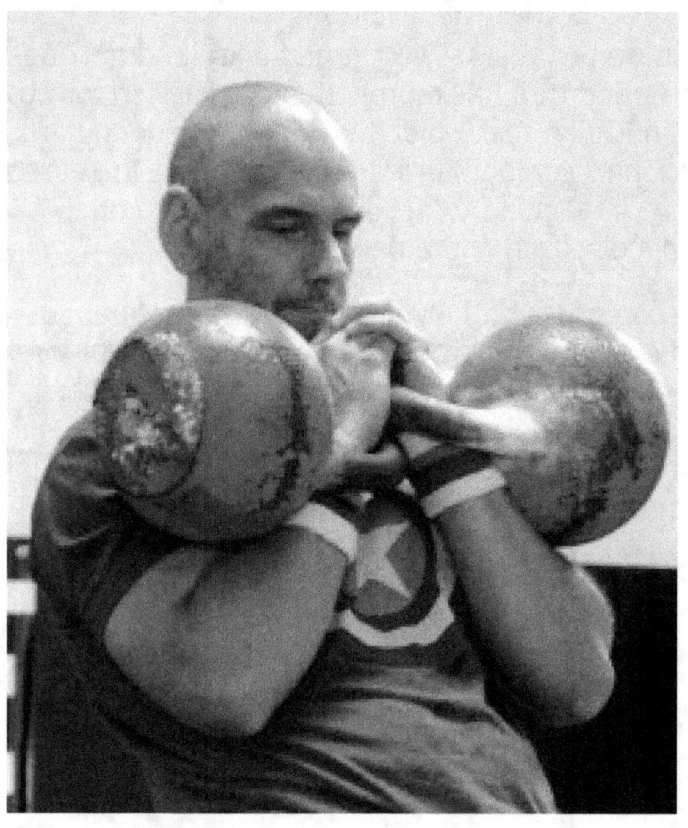

Like I said, I used to be fat, but now I'm not. I lost a lot of fat and a lot of weight, and I've kept it off for ten years now.

I lost 110 pounds, but it's really not that simple, although it sounds good in my elevator speech. I did lose 110lbs, but I've since added plenty of muscle, so today I'm back up to 200 pounds, yet leaner than when I was at my all-time low of 160.

In these ten years, I've learned a lot, and my quest to get fit and trim has morphed into a passion for fitness and nutrition that I didn't know I had hidden inside of me. That passion has led me to compete in Kettlebell Sport, in addition to becoming an IKFF certified kettlebell coach and a personal trainer.

As someone who's always been passionate about food and cooking, I'm proud to say that my weight loss journey has also spawned an interest in healthier eating and cooking, and together with my wife/coauthor, teach cooking classes for clients and friends. I'm also a Precision Nutrition Certified nutrition coach, and enjoy counseling others in their own weight loss journeys.

EatWellMoveWell.com

Facebook.com/TheFitInk

rdenzel@gmail.com

Twitter.com/RolandDenzel or @RolandDenzel

Galina Ivanova Denzel, NSCA-CPT, RES

Hi, my name is Galina Ivanova Denzel and I have spent the last 10 years of my life helping people get fit and healthy.

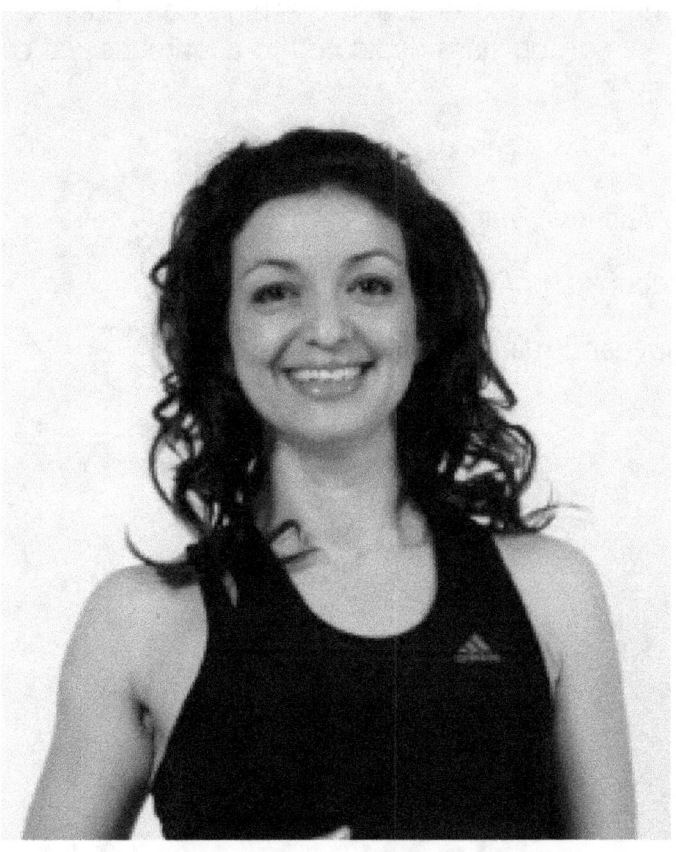

I am a Restorative Exercise™ Specialist (RES), personal trainer, nutrition coach, cookbook author and fitness writer. I specialize in working with people with special needs, from pregnancy and postnatal recovery, to low back and knee pain, diabetes or osteoporosis. I also work alongside clients who just want to lose some fat and get in shape. I have created a growing online consulting practice, and get to work with people all over the world! I also love seeing my local clients and teaching Core Connect – my own group class dedicated to alignment and core strength.

EatWellMoveWell.com

Facebook.com/TheFitInk

eatloveandtrain@gmail.com

Other Books by the Authors

Complete information on our books is available at EatWellMoveWell.com/Books

Man on Top: Lose Fat, Get Fit, and Control Your Weight for Life – A men's lifestyle, nutrition, and fitness manual. A guide for the busy man who doesn't want to change who he is just to get in shape.

The Real Food Reset – 30 days to lose weight, kick cravings, & feel great! Unlike a diet, a detox or a flush, The Real Food Reset develops healthy eating habits that become a platform for perfect health for the rest of your life. No weighing, measuring, or counting required!

Bigger • Stronger • Leaner – Time Tested Training based on the training of old time strongmen! The program for someone who's truly ready to train.

All you have to do is START! ...And Lose Weight Today – You've tried diet and exercise before, and you've always stopped. Diets are hard and restrictive, and who has time to go to the gym five times a week or train for a marathon just to slim down? You shouldn't have to change your whole life!

Thank you for reading!

If you enjoy the book, we'd love it if you write a review on Amazon, Apple, or Barnes & Noble!

It only takes a minute, it can be as short as 20 words, and it really does help others find us in a catalog of millions of books.

If you haven't subscribed to our newsletter, sign up today at EatWellMoveWell.com/contact.